I0416919

Your Free Gift

I wanted to show my appreciation for your purchase so I have put together a free gift for you!

Just visit the link below to download it now

http://newwheelpublishing.com/dashdiet/

I know you'll love this Gift.

Thanks!

Marie Harris

Contents

Introduction

Weight loss is important to a society that is increasingly sedentary and therefore reaching startling levels of obesity. With that obesity comes health problems, like high blood pressure.
Exercise is a strong step toward combatting health issues and the stigmas that come with being overweight.

However, exercise must be paired with a healthy diet in order to reach optimal success. There are the recommendations from the Food and Drug Administration via the food pyramid. These advise a 2,000 calorie daily diet and include certain servings from each of four food groups. This is helpful.

For those who already are suffering from high blood pressure and/or are overweight, a diet is advised by doctors. This is where the DASH Diet comes into play. This diet is based on the recommendations for healthy eating from the food pyramid. It outlines more precisely the best options for creating healthy meal plans and maintaining the diet long-term.

Chapter 1: What is the DASH Diet?

The DASH Diet is designed for one specific purpose, which is outlined in its full name

D: Dietary

A: Approaches to

S: Stop

H: Hypertension

This diet has the secondary benefit of weight loss and other health improvements because it focuses on fruits and vegetables and follows the Food Pyramid's outline for a 2,000 calorie daily intake (1).

The diet includes whole grains, poultry, fish and nuts so an emphasis on both protein and fiber exists. The importance of extra potassium, magnesium and calcium is also a strong thread to the DASH Diet, so low-fat dairy products are recommended. Limitations are placed on red meats and products that contain high levels of sugar, like sweets and sugary beverages.

.

A Diet Without Pills or Tricks

The DASH Diet is a reliable diet that is more easily maintained because it focuses on changing your eating habits and pairing that with more exercise. No pills, supplements or tricks are necessary to succeed with this diet. This also makes it easier to maintain, since no additional products need to be purchased.

Instead, it is a healthy way of living that helps you lengthen your life expectancy while losing weight and finding more pleasure in daily life.

Chapter 2: The DASH Diet: Effectiveness

In January of 2014, the DASH Diet was named the best overall diet for lowering weight and blood pressure and for lower cholesterol as well.

According to US News & World Report (2), the DASH Diet is the best diet overall because of its focus on fruits, vegetables and fish. The plant-based diet is also a high-ranking choice for people following Weight Watchers, since that program does not prohibit eating any specific group of foods.

This is the fourth year in a row the DASH Diet has received best overall diet honors. This shows the longevity of the diet's success. It also shows that people find it works and can be maintained in order to maintain the results that are desired.

Weight Loss

The DASH Diet's main focus is not to lose weight. Instead, it is meant to decrease hypertension. Therefore, the diet is based on 2,000 calories per day, which is what the Daily Food Pyramid already advises. If you can live by this diet for its intended purpose of decreasing hypertension and decrease caloric intake to 1,600 or less per day, the likelihood of losing weight increases drastically (3).

Lowering Blood Pressure

The DASH Diet is also helpful because it requires a reduction of the sodium in your diet to less than 2,300 milligrams per day. This helps avoid hypertension, or high blood pressure. If someone who already suffers from hypertension, this diet can help decrease the effects and bring your blood pressure to a more manageable level (1).

Chapter 3: Using the DASH Diet for weight loss

It is important to understand the DASH Diet was not created for weight loss purposes. However, if you begin with the effort to eat healthy and meet the calorie requirements, then aim for a caloric deficit each day (eating less than the recommended daily limit of 2,000 calories), then weight loss can be achieved.

The primary focus of this diet is less fat and sodium while eating a more balanced diet. This is a first step toward weight loss, because you eliminate the foods higher in calories and worse for your system.

Teenage Girls and Weight Loss

While not ideal to study teenagers who are still growing in terms of weight loss, this study shows how the diet is more a method to create and maintain a healthy lifestyle.

A study completed by Boston University Medical Center staff shows that the DASH Diet helps teenage girls avoid obesity simply by eating more fruits and vegetables and opting for low-fat dairy products (4).

The study followed almost 3,000 teenage girls and found that those who ate a diet closest to that recommended by the DASH Diet had the lowest Body Mass Index, or BMI. This study followed the youngsters, starting at age nine or 10, for a period of 10 years.

Chapter 4: Your weekly diet plan

Making a daily plan for the DASH Diet means meeting the recommendations for a certain number of servings of different food types.

The recommendation follows:

- Whole grains (6 to 8 servings a day)
- Vegetables (4 to 5 servings a day)
- Fruits (4 to 5 servings a day)
- Low-fat or fat-free milk and milk products (2 to 3 servings a day)
- Lean meats, poultry and fish (6 or fewer servings a day)
- Nuts, seeds and beans (4 to 5 servings a week)
- Fats and oils (2 to 3 servings a day)
- Sweets, preferably low-fat or fat-free (5 or fewer a week)
- Sodium (no more than 2,300 mg a day) (1)

Following these guidelines means a six-week plan must stay consistent, yet it must contain variety so you are likely to stay interested and not go off-diet.

Chapter 8 includes many healthy recipes that can be intermingled to reach the recommended servings of each category in the diet.

The Mayo Clinic (5) has created sample menus for individuals who need help starting out in the DASH Diet. Below is a three-day sample of menus, divided into each meal and complete with nutrient analysis.

Day 1 menu

Breakfast

1 small whole-wheat bagel with 2 tablespoons peanut butter (no salt added)
1 medium orange
1 cup fat-free milk
Decaffeinated coffee

Lunch

Spinach salad made with:

- 4 cups of fresh spinach leaves
- 1 sliced pear
- 1/2 cup canned mandarin orange sections
- 1/3 cup slivered almonds
- 2 tablespoons reduced-fat red wine vinaigrette

12 reduced-sodium wheat crackers
1 cup fat-free milk

Dinner

Herb-crusted baked cod, 3 ounces
1/2 cup brown rice pilaf
1/2 cup fresh green beans, steamed
1 small sourdough roll
2 teaspoon trans-free margarine
1 cup fresh berries with chopped mint
Herbal iced tea

Snack (anytime)

1 cup fat-free, low-calorie yogurt
4 vanilla wafers

Day 1 nutrient analysis

Calories	1,810	Cholesterol	
Protein	86 grams (g)	Sodium	
Carbohydrate	247 g	Fiber	
Total fat	53 g	Potassium	
Saturated fat	7 g	Calcium	
Monounsaturated fat	23 g		

Day 1 DASH servings

Grains and grain products	7
Vegetables	5
Fruits	5
Dairy foods (low-fat or fat-free)	3
Meats, poultry and fish	3
Nuts, seeds and dry beans	2
Fats and oils	3
Sweets	1

Day 2 menu

Breakfast

1 cup fresh mixed fruits, such as melons, banana, apple and berries, topped with 1 cup fat-free, low-calorie vanilla-flavored yogurt and 1/3 cup walnuts
1 bran muffin
1 teaspoon trans-free margarine
1 cup fat-free milk
Herbal tea

Lunch

Curried chicken wrap made with:

- 1 medium whole-wheat tortilla
- 2/3 cup cooked, chopped chicken, about 3 ounces
- 1/2 cup chopped apple
- 2 tablespoons fat-free mayonnaise*
- 1/2 teaspoon curry powder

1/2 cup, or about 8, raw baby carrots
1 cup fat-free milk

Dinner	1 cup cooked whole-wheat spaghetti with 1 cup marinara sauce, no added salt 2 cups mixed salad greens 1 tablespoon low-fat Caesar dressing 1 whole-wheat roll 1 teaspoon trans-free margarine 1 nectarine Sparkling water
Snack (anytime)	Trail mix made with:

- 1/4 cup raisins
- 1 ounce, or about 22, unsalted mini twist pretzels
- 2 tablespoons sunflower seeds

*Fat-free spreads still have calories so count as 1 fat serving.

Day 2 nutrient analysis

Calories	1,953	Cholesterol	85 mg
Protein	89 g	Sodium	1,816 mg
Carbohydrate	280 g	Fiber	43 g
Total fat	53 g	Potassium	3,295 mg
Saturated fat	6 g	Calcium	1,267 mg
Monounsaturated fat	19 g		

Day 2 DASH servings

Grains and grain products	7
Vegetables	6
Fruits	5
Dairy foods (low-fat or fat-free)	3
Meats, poultry and fish	3
Nuts, seeds and dry beans	2
Fats and oils	3
Sweets	0

Day 3 menu

Breakfast

1 cup old-fashioned cooked oatmeal* topped with 1 teaspoon cinnamon
1 slice whole-wheat toast
1 teaspoon trans-free margarine
1 banana
1 cup fat-free milk

Lunch

Tuna salad made with:

- 1/2 cup drained, unsalted water-packed tuna, 3 ounces
- 2 tablespoons fat-free

mayonnaise

- 15 grapes
- 1/4 cup diced celery
- Served on top of 2 cups romaine lettuce

8 Melba toast crackers
1 cup fat-free milk

Dinner

Beef and vegetable kebab, made with:

- 3 ounces of beef
- 1 cup of peppers, onions, mushrooms and cherry tomatoes

1 cup cooked wild rice
1/3 cup pecans
2 pineapple rings

Cran-raspberry spritzer made with:

- 4 ounces cran-raspberry juice
- 4 to 8 ounces sparkling water

Snack (anytime)

1 cup light yogurt
1 peach

*To further reduce sodium, don't add salt when cooking the oatmeal.

Day 3 nutrient analysis

Calories	1,834	Cholesterol	98 mg
Protein	105 g	Sodium	984 mg
Carbohydrate	250 g	Fiber	28 g
Total fat	46 g	Potassium	4,215 mg
Saturated fat	8 g	Calcium	1,122 mg
Monounsaturated fat	21 g		

Day 3 DASH servings

Grains and grain products	6
Vegetables	5
Fruits	5
Dairy foods (low-fat or fat-free)	3
Meats, poultry and fish	6
Nuts, seeds and dry beans	1
Fats and oils	2
Sweets	0

(5)

Chapter 5: Top recipes for your plan

BREAKFAST

RECIPE: Granola Oatmeal

- ¼ teaspoon of salt
- ¼ cup of honey
- ½ teaspoon of vanilla extract
- 1/3 cup of sliced almonds
- ½ cup of whole wheat flour
- 1 ½ cups of regular oats (uncooked)
- 2 tablespoons of melted light butter

1) Get a small bowl, and stir together honey, light butter and vanilla extract.
2) Get a large bowl and stir together oats, almonds, salt and flour.
3) Add the honey mixture into the oats mixture and stir until combined.
4) In a greased baking sheet, spread the oat mixture and bake and stir often at 350 degrees for about 20 minutes.

RECIPE: Flatbread Club Sandwich

- 24 large beaten eggs
- 1 ½ cups of water
- 2 teaspoon of dried thyme
- 2 teaspoon of onion powder
- 12 8-9 inches of round or oblong flatbreads
- 18 ounces of cheddar cheese (shredded)
- 12 ounce of Canadian bacon
- 12 ounce of turkey deli meat slices
- 12 cooked, halved, bacon slices
- 1 teaspoon of pepper (cracked)

1) Blend eggs with water and spices.
2) For each sandwich you'll make pour, 2/3 cup of the egg mixtures into a coated non-stick pan. Cook it omelette style, until its firm with no visible liquid egg.
3) Add omelette into a horizontally positioned flatbread. Add layer of 1 ounce Canadian bacon, 1 ounce turkey, 2 halved bacon slices and 1 ½ ounce of cheddar cheese.
4) Fold flatbread in half.

RECIPE: Burrito for Breakfast

- 3 egg whites
- 1 egg
- 1 teaspoon of grape seed oil
- ¼ cup of diced onion
- ½ sliced red pepper
- 1 teaspoon of grape seed oil
- ¼ teaspoon of cumin
- ¼ diced avocado
- 1 tablespoon of chopped cilantro
- 1 tortilla rice
- Sea salt and pepper (to taste)

1) Heat grape seed oil in a frying pad then add onion and pepper. Quickly fry for 5 minutes or until vegetables are tender. Season with cumin, sea salt and pepper

2) Stir it with egg, scramble everything and cook for 4 minutes. Before eggs are cook or set, stir it with cilantro.

3) Turn off the heat and finish cooking the eggs from the heat of the pan.

4) Put the tortilla on an oven on low heat until each side is slightly charred

5) Fill the tortilla with the scramble and top it with the diced avocado, Cut the burrito in half and serve.

RECIPE: No Need to Bake Granola Bars

- 2 Cups of Oatmeal
- 2 ½ cups of toasted rice cereal
- ½ cup of raisins
- ½ cup of light corn syrup
- ½ cup of brown sugar
- ½ cup of peanut butter
- 1 tsp of vanilla

1) Combine the oatmeal, rice cereal and raisins in a mixing bowl and stir together.
2) Get a saucepan, put and mix together the brown sugar and corn syrup.
3) Turn heat into medium-high and stir the mixture until it boils. Remove saucepan from heat once the mixture is boiling
4) Put the peanut butter and vanilla into the sugar mixture and blend until it's smooth.
5) Pour the peanut butter mixture over the cereal and raisins and mix it well in the bowl
6) Place the mixture into a baking pan and let it cool.

RECIPE: Bacon and Cheese Omelette

- Canadian Style Bacon-1/2 cup
- Shredded Cheddar Cheese (reduced-fat)-1/2 cup
- No stick cooking spray
- 16 oz each of egg beaters original (1 carton)
- 1/8 tsp of ground black pepper

1) In a bowl, combine the Egg beaters and ground black pepper then set aside.
2) Get a frying pan and spray it with the no stick cooking spray. Set it over medium heat and add bacon. Cook until Canadian bacon is browned and remove from the frying pan and set aside.
3) Add ½ of the Egg beater mixture into the frying pan and cook until the edges are set. Tilt the frying pan while

gently lifting the edges for the uncooked eggs to run underneath.

4) Put or sprinkle half of Canadian bacon and half of cheddar cheese into half of the cooked eggs beaters. Fold over and slide omelette into plate. Repeat up to for servings.

RECIPE: Casserole made with sweet potatoes

- 16 oz each of egg beaters original (1 carton)
- 3 Chopped Sausage patties
- 3 cups of frozen sweet potato cubes
- No stick cooking spray
- 1 cup of low fat cottage cheese
- ½ cup of reduced/low fat cheddar cheese (shredded)
- ½ cup of fat free milk
- ¼ cup of maple syrup
- ½ tsp of salt
- 1/8 tsp of ground black pepper

1) Preheat and oven to 176 Celsius or 350 degrees Fahrenheit and spray a baking dish with the no stick cooking spray and set aside.
2) Mix the Eggs with maple syrup, salt, ground black pepper and milk in a bowl. After mixing, add the sausage patties, sweet potatoes, ¼ cup of cheddar cheese, and low fat cottage cheese. Stir to combine.
3) Pour the mixture into the dish and baked for at least 75 minutes. Get the remaining ¼ cup of cheddar cheese and sprinkle it into the dish and bake until the cheese melts.

RECIPE: Green smoothie on the go

- 1 Banana
- ½ tsp of vanilla
- ¼ cup of non-fat yogurt
- ¾ cup of mango (frozen)

- ¼ cup of oats
- ½ cup of milk (fat-free)
- 1 cup of packed spinach

1) Put the ½ cup of milk, ¼ cup of non-fat yogurt and ¼ cup of oats in a blender and blend for 15-20 seconds(High speed)
2) Add ¾ cup of mango, 1 cup of packed spinach, pour ½ tsp of vanilla, and place the banana.
3) Blend everything until smooth.

LUNCH

RECIPE: Pizza made of pita breads

- Pita bread (whole wheat)
- ¼ cup of tomato sauce
- ½ cup of mozzarella cheese (Less sodium)
- Your vegetable of choice

1) Preheat an oven to 350 degrees.
2) Split the whole wheat pita bread halfway and put the mozzarella cheese, tomato sauce and your choice of veggies.
3) Wrap the pita bread in an aluminum foil and bake until the cheese melts (around 10 minutes).

RECIPE: Easy to make chicken salad

- 3 ¼ cups of skinless chicken breast
- ¼ cup of chopped celery
- 1/8 teaspoon of salt
- 3 tablespoon of low-fat mayonnaise
- 1 tablespoon of lemon juice
- ½ teaspoon of onion powder

1) Cut the chicken into small cubes then, bake then refrigerate

2) In a bowl, combine the ingredients and add the refrigerated (chilled) chicken and mix well.

RECIPE: The Tuna Melt

- 3 oz low/reduced-fat grated cheese
- 2 whole wheat muffins
- 6 oz of drained tuna packed in water
- 1/4 cup of onion (chopped)
- 1/3 cup of celery (chopped)
- ¼ cup of low fat salad dressing

1) Combine/Mix tuna, 1/3 cup of celery, ¼ cup of onion and the ¼ cup low fat salad dressing. (Optional: season salt and pepper)
2) Toast wheat muffin in half and split side up on oven and put ¼ of tuna mixture on top.
3) Heat or broil for 3-4 minutes then top it with grated cheese. Heat for another minute or until the cheese is melted.

RECIPE: HOT star shrimp

- 1 pound peeled shrimp (raw)
- 4 tablespoon of tomato paste
- 3 teaspoon of water
- 1 teaspoon of garlic (minced)
- 1 teaspoon of olive oil
- 1 teaspoon of chilli powder
- 1 teaspoon of chopped fresh oregano
- No stick cooking spray

1) Wash the shrimp and dry with paper towel. Put on a plate and set aside
2) Mix the tomato paste, water and olive oil.
3) Add the minced garlic, oregano and chilli powder into the tomato paste mixture.
4) For every shrimp, put the mixture onto both sides.
5) Take the grill rack and spray it with the no stick cooking

spray (please take note that you spray away from the heat of the grill) then place the rack 6 inches from the heat.
6) Place shrimp and turn it every 3 minutes. Watch as the cooking time depends on the heat of your grill.

RECIPE: Delicious pork chops

- 6 center-cut pork chops,
- ½ inch thick of liquid egg white
- 1 cup of fat-free evaporated milk
- ¾ cup of cornflake crumbs
- ¼ cup of breadcrumbs
- 4 teaspoon of paprika
- 2 teaspoon of oregano
- ¾ teaspoon of chilli powder
- ½ teaspoon of garlic powder
- ½ teaspoon of ground black pepper
- 1/8 teaspoon of cayenne pepper
- 1/8 teaspoon of dry mustard
- ½ teaspoon of salt

1) Preheat your oven to 375 °F or 190 degrees Celsius.
2) Trim fat pork chops
3) Mix/beat the egg white and evaporated milk. Place pork chops in milk mixture. Turn it once after 5 minutes.
4) Mix the crumbs, breadcrumbs, salt and other spices.
5) Spray your pan with a cooking spray.
6) Remove pork chops from your milk mixture and coat it with the crumbs mixture.
7) Place the pork chops in your pan and bake at 375 °F for 15-20 minutes.
8) Turn pork chops and bake for another 15-20 minutes or until pork is cooked.

RECIPE: Brown rice with Skinless and Boneless Chicken

- 1 cup of chopped onions

- ¼ cup of green peppers
- 2 teaspoon of vegetable oil
- 1 tomato sauce (8oz)
- 1 teaspoon of chopped parsley
- ½ teaspoon of black pepper
- 1 ¼ teaspoon of minced garlic
- Cooked rice in unsalted water (5 cups)
- 3 ½ cups of diced and cooked chicken (bone and skin removed)

1) Quickly fry the green peppers and chopped onions in oil for about 5 minutes.
2) Quickly add the other spices and tomato sauce, heat thorough.
3) Add the cooked rice and heat through.

RECIPE: Savory Baked Fish

- 1 pound of your favorite fillet fish
- 1 tablespoon of olive oil
- 1 teaspoon of salt free spicy seasoning
- Cooking oil spray
- Rice (Optional)

1) Preheat your oven to 350°F.
2) Spray your pan with cooking oil spray.
3) Wash and dry fish using paper towel. Place fish in a dish and mix the olive oil and spicy seasoning lightly over fish.
4) Bake for 15-20 minutes uncovered
5) Serve with rice.

DINNER

RECIPE: Spicy Rellenos

- 3 large (any color) halved bell peppers

- 2 eggs
- 4 tbsp of mashed avocado
- 1 1/2 C reduced fat Mexican style shredded cheese
- 1/2 C plain non-fat Greek yogurt
- 1/2 C plain non-fat Greek yogurt

Legend:

*tbsp- tablespoon, *C- cups

1) At 350 F, preheat the oven. Wash the bell peppers and cut into halves. Remove the seeds and cores from the peppers. Place the pepper halves in a 7.5 x 11 inch baking pan and fit it snuggly to prevent spillage when filling. Set aside afterwards.
2) Whisk the remaining ingredients in a large bowl together until well combined. Distribute mixture evenly into each of the bell pepper halves, filling it fully without spilling out.
3) For about 30-45 minutes, place pan in oven and cook, or up until the cheese is golden brown, the egg cooked and the toothpick inserted comes out. Top with salsa and serve.

RECIPE: Lean Beef Burgers

- 1 pound 95% lean ground beef
- 2 tbsp quick-cooking oats
- 1/2 tsp steak seasoning blend
- Whole wheat hamburger buns, split
- Slices of low-fat cheese (Cheddar or American)
- Toppings:
  Lettuce leaf, tomato slices (optional)

*tbsp –tablespoon

*tsp- teaspoon

1) Seal oats securely in a food-safe plastic bag squeezing

out excess air. Use rolling pin to roll over bag and crush oats to a fine consistency.

2) In a large bowl, mix lightly but thoroughly the ground beef, oats, and steak seasoning blend. Shape lightly into 1/2-inch patties.

3) Place patties on grid over medium with ash-covered coals. Grill for about 11-13 minutes over medium heat on a preheated grill (7-8 minutes) while covered until the instant-read thermometer which is inserted horizontally into the center registers to 160°F while turning occasionally.

4) With lettuce and tomato, line the bottom of each bun, if desired; top with burger and cheese slice and then close the sandwiches.

RECIPE: Jamaican Spiced Chicken with Mango Topper

- For Mango Topper

  2 peeled ripe mangos, pitted and cut into 1/4-inch dice
  1/4 cup of lime juice
  2 tablespoon of brown sugar
  1/2 teaspoon of crushed red pepper
  1/4 teaspoon of garlic powder
  1/4 teaspoon of cinnamon
  1/4 teaspoon of ground allspice

- For Chicken

  4 slightly flattened boneless, skinless chicken breasts (about 1 1/2 pounds)
  2 tablespoon of Jamaican jerk seasoning blend
  1 halved lime

1) In a medium bowl, mix the mango, lime juice, brown sugar, red pepper, garlic powder, cinnamon and allspice and then set aside.

2) Rinse chicken and pat dry then sprinkle the jerk seasoning on both sides and let it stand for 10 minutes.

For about 5 to 7 minutes over medium heat, cook each side of the chicken on a well-oiled grill, or until chicken is cooked through.

3) After removing from grill, squeeze lime halves over chicken and serve with the mango topper.

RECIPE: Shrimp Pasta

- 1 ¼ cup of fresh asparagus, sliced into 1-inch lengths (about 1/2 pound)
- 1 ½ cup (12oz) of whole wheat penne pasta
- 1 cup green peas, fresh or frozen
- 2 teaspoon of olive oil
- 1 tablespoon of minced garlic
- 1/8 teaspoon of crushed red pepper
- 1 pound peeled and medium shrimp
- 1/2 cup of thinly sliced green onion
- 2 teaspoon of fresh lemon juice
- 1 tablespoon of fresh parsley (chopped)
- 1/3 cup of grated cheese
- 1/2 teaspoon of salt
- Fresh ground black pepper

1) Boil 6 quart pot of water and add asparagus. For about 4 minutes, cook until tender-crisp. Using a slotted spoon, transfer to a bowl.

2) Cook and add the pasta following the package directions. Add the peas in the last 2 minutes of cooking. Along with the peas, drain the pasta and reserve with the asparagus in a bowl.

3) In a 12-inch non-stick skillet, heat the olive oil over medium heat. Then, add the minced garlic and crushed red pepper and for about 1 minute, cook, stirring, until fragrant.

4) Add the shrimp and for about 2 minutes cook it on each side. Add the green onion, lemon juice, parsley, vegetables and cheese with the pasta then toss to coat

and season with salt and fresh ground black pepper to taste.

RECIPE: Chilli Loaded Sweet Potato

- 4 medium sized sweet potatoes
- ½ cup of fat free Greek yogurt or light sour cream
- 1 teaspoon of taco seasoning (low sodium)
- 1 teaspoon olive oil
- 1 or ½ cup of diced red pepper
- ½ diced red onion
- 1 teaspoon chilli powder
- ½ teaspoon of Paprika
- ½ teaspoon of Cumin
- A pinch of salt
- 1 1/3 cup of canned sodium black beans (rinsed and drained)
- ½ cup of reduced fat Mexican cheese blend
- ¼ cup chopped scallions or cilantro
- ½ cup salsa (optional)

1) With a fork, poke holes in the potato and cook on your microwave's setting for potatoes until they are soft and cooked through (about 8-10 minutes on high for 4 potatoes). If a microwave is not available, in 400°F, bake in the oven for about 45 minutes. Mix the yogurt and taco seasoning well in a small bowl.
2) In a medium pot, heat the oil over medium heat then add peppers, onions, chilli powder, paprika, cumin and salt and for about 5 minutes, cook until the onions have caramelized slightly.
3) Add black beans, stir to combine and heat through for another 5 minutes.

4) In a lengthwise manner, slice the potato down the middle or use a fork to pierce the skin. Top with 2 tablespoon of shredded cheese, 1/3 cup of black bean mixture, 2 tablespoon of Greek yogurt mixture and 2 tablespoon of salsa.

RECIPE: Vegetable Pie Topped with Oregon Hazelnut

- 1 cups of chopped fresh broccoli
- 1 cups of sliced fresh cauliflower
- 2 cups of chopped fresh spinach
- 1/2 cups of chopped onion
- 1/4 cups chopped green pepper
- 1 cups of cheddar cheese, grated (4 oz.)
- 1 cups of coarsely chopped Oregon hazelnuts
- 1 ½ cups non-fat milk
- 1 cups baking mix
- 4 eggs
- 1/4 teaspoon pepper

1) For about 5 minutes, pre-cook broccoli and cauliflower until almost tender and drain well.
2) Mix the broccoli, cauliflower, onion, spinach, green pepper and cheese. In well-greased 8-inch pie pans, divide into two then top it with Oregon hazelnuts.
3) Beat together milk, baking mix, eggs, garlic and pepper and then pour over vegetable mixture.
4) Bake at 400 degrees Fahrenheit for 35 to 40 minutes or until the color turns into golden brown.
5) Before cutting, allow to stand for 5 minutes.

RECIPE: Chicken with Cranberry sauce

- 1 pound chicken breasts (skinless and boneless)
- 1 teaspoon of butter
- ¼ teaspoon of ground black pepper

- ¾ cup of whole cranberry sauce
- ¼ cup of chilli sauce
- ¼ cup of apple juice
- 1 teaspoon of brown sugar

1) Slightly pound chicken and sprinkle with pepper.
2) Brown the chicken in butter in a large pan.
3) Add the remaining ingredients and for about 15 minutes, simmer while covered.
4) As you remove the lid, boil until the sauce is desired thickness.

DESSERT

RECIPE: Cheesecake with Lemon Zest

- 2 tablespoon of cold water
- 1 envelope of gelatin (unflavoured)
- 2 tablespoon of lemon juice
- 1/2 cup of heated skim milk
- Egg substitute = 1 egg or 2 eggs
- 1/4 cup of sugar
- 1 teaspoon of vanilla
- 2 cups of cottage cheese (low-fat)
- Lemon zest (optional)

1) In blender container, mix water, gelatin and lemon juice.
2) For 1 to 2 minutes, process on low speed to soften gelatin. Add hot milk while processing to dissolve gelatin.
3) Put the egg substitute along with sugar, vanilla and cheese into blender container and process it on

high speed.

4)   When already smooth, pour into 9" pie plate or round flat dish. Refrigerate for to 2 to 3 hours.

5)   Top with grated lemon zest just before serving if you wish to do so.

RECIPE: Almond-Apricot Biscotti

- 3/4 cup of whole-wheat flour
- 3/4 cup of all-purpose plain flour
- 1/4 cup of brown sugar, packed firmly
- 1 teaspoon of baking powder
- 2 lightly beaten eggs
- 2 tablespoon of 1% low-fat milk
- 2 tablespoon of canola oil
- 2 tablespoon of dark honey
- 1/2 teaspoon of almond extract
- 2/3 cup of dried apricots, chopped
- 1/4 cup of almonds, coarsely chopped

1) At the temperature of 350 F, Preheat the oven.
2) Mix the flours, brown sugar and baking powder in a large bowl and whisk to blend. Into the mixture, put the eggs, milk, canola oil, honey and almond extract. Up until the dough begins to stick, keep stirring with a wooden spoon. Add the chopped apricots and almonds and mix with floured hands until the dough is well blended.
3) On a long sheet of plastic wrap, place the dough and shape by hand into a 12-inch flattened log, about 3 inches wide and an inch high.
4) Onto a non-stick baking sheet, lift the plastic wrap to invert the dough and for about 25 to 30 minutes, bake until lightly browned. Cool for 10 minutes after transferring to another baking sheet. Just keep the oven set at 350 F.
5) Cut the cooled log on a crosswise with a serrated knife

on the diagonal into 24 slices 1/2 inch wide. Cut-side down, arrange the slices on the baking sheet.

6) For about 15 to 20 minutes, return to the oven and bake until crisp. Let it cool completely after transferring to a wire rack and store in an airtight container.

RECIPE: Rice Pudding topped with Almond

- 3 cups of almond milk
- 1 cup of white rice
- 4 tablespoon of sugar
- 1 teaspoon of vanilla
- 1/4 teaspoon of almond extract
- 4 tablespoon of toasted almonds (optional)

1) In a 2-3 quart saucepan, combine the almond with the milk and rice and bring to a boil.
2) For 1/2 hour, reduce heat and simmer with the lid on until the rice is soft.
3) Mix in the sugar, vanilla, almond extract and cinnamon.
4) Serve warm and sprinkle toasted almonds on top.
5) Leftovers must be refrigerated within 2 hours.

RECIPE: Cream Cheese-topped Red Velvet Pancakes

- For Cream Cheese Topping:
  60 mL of 1/3 less fat cream cheese
  3 tablespoons of plain fat free yogurt
  3 tablespoons of honey
  1 tablespoon of fat-free milk
- Pancakes:
  ½ cup of white whole wheat flour
  ½ cup of unbleached all-purpose flour
  2 ¼ teaspoon of baking powder
  ½ tablespoon of cocoa powder (unsweetened)
  ¼ teaspoon of salt
  ¼ cup of sugar
  1 egg, large

1 cup+ 2 tablespoon of fat-free milk
1 teaspoon of vanilla
½ teaspoon of red paste food coloring

1. Set aside the mixed cream cheese topping ingredients. In a large bowl, combine the flours, baking powder, cocoa powder, sugar, and salt. In another bowl, use milk to dissolve the food colouring; whisk in egg and vanilla.

2. Mix both wet and dry ingredients but make sure that you don't over mix them. Just mix until there's no more dry spots.

3. Prepare a non-stick griddle pan and heat on medium-low heat. After heating, coat lightly with oil by spraying and pour ¼ cup of the pancake batter onto the pan.

4. Flip the pancake when it starts to bubble and the edges begin to set. Do the same with the remainder of the batter.

5. Place 2 pancakes on each plate and then top it with about 2 ½ tablespoons of the cream cheese topping.

RECIPE: Moist Fig Bars

- 2 cups of stemmed, chopped dried figs
- ½ cups of chopped walnuts
- 1/3 cups of sugar
- ¼ cups of orange juice
- 2 tablespoon of hot water
- ½ cups of margarine, softened
- 1 cups of packed brown sugar
- 1 egg, large
- 1 ½ cups of all-purpose flour

- ½ teaspoon of baking soda
- 1 ¼ cups of old fashioned rolled oats

1. At 350 F, preheat the oven. Lightly spray oil on a 9x13-inch baking pan.
2. In a mixing bowl, put together and mix the figs, walnuts, sugar, orange juice and hot water; set aside afterwards. Beat the margarine and brown sugar together until creamy and add the egg and mix until smooth.
3. Combine flour and baking soda, stir into the egg mixture and blend in oats to make soft dough. For topping, reserve one cup of dough.
4. Press the remaining dough with floured fingertips into a thin layer of dough on the bottom of the baking pan. Over the dough, spread the fig mixture evenly and pat firmly. By teaspoonful's, crumble reserved dough over top to allow fig mixture to show.
5. Bake for half an hour or until golden brown and cool completely in a baking pan. Cut into 1 x 3 inch bars. Leftovers should be refrigerated within 2 hours.

RECIPE: Carrot Cookies

- 1 teaspoon of vanilla
- 1 cup of flour
- 1 cup of whole wheat flour
- 1 teaspoon of baking soda
- 1 teaspoon of baking powder
- 1⁄4 teaspoon of salt
- 1 teaspoon of ground cinnamon
- 1⁄2 teaspoon of ground nutmeg
- 1⁄2 teaspoon of ground ginger
- 2 cups of old-fashioned rolled oats (raw)
- 1 1⁄2 cups of finely grated carrots (about 3 large carrots)
- 1 cup of raisins or golden raisins

- 1 Egg
- 1 cup of white sugar
- Oil

1) At 350 F, preheat the oven.
2) Combine/Mix the sugar
3) Combine these four ingredients thoroughly: sugar, oil, applesauce, eggs, and vanilla
4) Mix dry ingredients together and blend into wet mixture.
5) Mix in the raisins and carrots.
6) On a greased cookie sheet, drop by teaspoonful and bake until golden brown for about 12-15 minutes. Store the cookies in airtight container afterwards.

RECIPE: Berry Banana Ice Cream

- 3 frozen bananas cut into 1-inch pieces
- 1 cup of frozen berries
- 1/2 cup of non-fat milk
- 1 1/2 teaspoon of vanilla extract

1) Peel and slice bananas and put them in the freezer over-night. After at least 8 hours, remove the bananas from the freezer and add them to a food processor.
2) Add the milk and vanilla and process for 1-2 minutes. Stop processor and scrape down the sides once banana is broken up.
3) Continue to process only stopping as needed to scrape down the sides of the bowl until it reaches the consistency of soft serve ice cream.
4) Pulse the berries in until they are in pieces and incorporated into the banana mixture. Serve immediately afterwards.

Your Free Gift

I wanted to show my appreciation for your purchase so I have put together a free gift for you!

Just visit the link below to download it now

http://newwheelpublishing.com/dashdiet/

I know you'll love this Gift.

Thanks!

Marie Harris

www.ingramcontent.com/pod-product-compliance
Lightning Source LLC
Chambersburg PA
CBHW071327310526
45789CB00016B/1760